# ANCIENT EGYPTIAN SECRETS FOR HEALTH

*MOHAMED MALAH*

# Table of Contents


Chapter 1. Introduction To Ancient Egyptian

Chapter 2. Agriculture In The Era Of Ancient Egyptians

Chapter 3. Return To The Peasants' Food

Chapter 4. Vegetables

Chapter 5. Fruits

Chapter 6. Herbs

Chapter 7. Honey

Chapter 8. important Prescriptions In Ancient Egyptians

Chapter 9. Aromatherapy

Chapter 10. Face And Skin Care

Chapter 11. Medical Papyrus Discovered

About The Author

# CHAPTER 1. INTRODUCTION TO ANCIENT EGYPTIAN

The ancient Egyptian society consists of a group of different classes, the highest one was the pharaoh and his family, then followed by the ministers, the high priests, the scribes, the rulers of the provinces, small staff, merchants, and craftsmen. Now let's walk around in the life of the ancient Egyptian family to learn about the role of father, mother, and children in terms of their rights, duties, housing, clothing, customs, traditions and entertainment.

## FAMILY

The ancient Egyptian family consisted of father, mother and children, each of them had a role to play. The father was the head of the family, he provides them with their needs, protects them and has the right to be obeyed and respected by The wife and children. The mother occupied an important position in the family. She supervised the affairs of the house from cleaning, arranging and cooking. She also took care of her children, helped her husband in some work, and had the right to inherit, sell and purchase. The children were raised by their parents who wanted to teach them good morals and various sciences, the children were keen to succeed in their studies and respect their parents, help them in their work, and care of their graves after their death.

## HOUSING AND ESTABLISHMENT

The old Egyptian houses were characterized by simplicity, it was consisted of one or two floors with one or two rooms, it was constructed of bricks, except for the openings of doors and columns, it was constructed of stones. The houses of the rich were bigger and surrounded with beautiful gardens, the walls were decorated with ornaments and various inscriptions. The Palace of Pharaoh was the ideal in the height and luxury.

## FURNITURE

The houses were full of beds, pillows, benches, wooden boxes for keeping clothes, tables, food and water containers, furniture varied from house to house according to the living conditions of the family

## CLOTHING

The old Egyptian was interested in his clothes, which differed from one class to another according to the living conditions of each class. The public clothes of the people were made of linen, but the clothes of the rich and the pharaoh were made of silk and embroidered in gold and silver.

## ADORNMENT

The ancient Egyptians liked to adorn themselves, using chains, earrings, bracelets, perfumes, combs, henna, kohl and rings

## CUSTOMS AND TRADITIONS

The traditions of ancient Egyptian had changed by time. At the beginning he was eating his food on mats, then he knew the low tables then he also knew the high tables with the seats. He also knew the three meals system in one day, washing hands before and after meals. He does not enter the houses until he has been given permission.

## ENTERTAINMENT

The life of the ancient Egyptians wasn't that serious as they often make use of some methods of entertainment such as fishing and hunting quails, pigeons, ducks, fish, crocodiles, deer and lions

## SPORTS GAMES

The old Egyptian knew many games to entertain himself, such as the game of shooting on a wooden block, wrestling, fencing, weight lifting, ball game, stick game, ring, and hide face.

## MUSIC AND SINGING

The ancient Egyptians knew the music and loved it, such as playing the flute, drums and singing individually or in group.

## HOLIDAYS AND CELEBRATIONS

The ancient Egyptians celebrated their important seasons and festivals such as the Spring Festival, New Year's Eve, the Day of God Amun, the God Osiris, the day of the inauguration of Pharaoh as president, the feast of victory, Easter, flood feast, the Festival of Sacrifice.

## PHARAOH

The Pharaoh was also the prime minister and he has more than one minister, the most important one who is responsible for administration and money. He is the most reliable person after Pharaoh. There was also a government council of 10 people who help the Pharaoh in making decisions.

## THE FARMERS

The farmers gained great importance during the era of Egyptians. Their goal was to plant all the banks of the

Nile River and to take care of its surroundings after any flooding, as they were like a tour guide who knows all the details of those lands.

## THE WRITER

The writer of the ancient Egyptians was of great importance and was responsible for various jobs according to his degree, such as drafting letters or teaching illiterate citizens, as he was respected by all because of his knowledge, and senior writers did not pay taxes

## CATS

Cats had a special position for Egyptians because they hunt rats, snakes. Also, they were associated with Bastet God, when a cat died, the owner shaves his eyebrows and declare mourning for 70 days.

## DWARFS

*DWARFS IN ANCIENT EGYPT ARE TWO TYPES:*

The first type is the African dwarf who was brought by the ancient Egyptian during his trade with Nubia and the land of Punt, their role was to dance in the royal palace to bring pleasure to the heart of the king. The first dwarf was brought from the land of Punt during the reign of King Isesi of the Fifth Dynasty

The second type is the Egyptian dwarfs who were famous for the jewelry industry. Although they suffered from physical deformity, they were characterized by a large head, a natural trunk, and short limbs, but they were famous for the jewelry industry in ancient Egypt due to the small limbs that enabled them to easily shape jewelry and distinguish them from others. They have a picture on the walls of the Mereruka cemetery in Saqqara

## DWARF SNAPE

Snape was a minister in the fifth family from the history of the Pharaohs, who ruled Egypt until the last ruler, he did not care about his defect and he was proud of himself, especially as he is married to one of the princesses and there is a statue in the Egyptian Museum sitting with his wife, She wears a black wig with a long white robe and a smile on her face that expresses the satisfaction of the woman and puts her hand on him with pride, love and a statue of their children under her husband's feet.

# Chapter 2. Agriculture In The Era Of Ancient Egyptians

The abundance of Nile water and fertile soil helped to grow many food crops such as peas, garlic, lettuce, onions and fruits such as grapes, figs, pomegranates, watermelons and dates, which were the fruit of most of the population.

The ancient Egyptian was in charge of his health, and this appeared in artistic inscriptions as well as Pharaonic sculptures. The male enjoys strong bodies and women are keen to appear beautiful and graceful. The ancient Egyptians considered it is shameful for a man to love food greedily and that a little water was enough. Some men would recommend his sons Be humble with food, a few loaves of bread are enough for you today. If you do not know how to be jealous, fight your stomach

# Chapter 4. Vegetables

## Fava Beans

fava beans are one of the popular foods since the beginning of the Pharaonic era where it was eaten after cooking by burying it in the dust of the hot oven and saw on the walls of the tombs drawings of the agricultural crops that were offered to the god Amun Hummus was also used as a food after its treatment, as was the thermos, which was eaten after it was soaked in water and its salts were of great importance in many medicinal purposes for its usefulness in the treatment of constipation, diabetes

The ancient Egyptians also accepted to eat cowpea, peas for their food and health benefits, so fava beans became the main food of the ancient Egyptians until the people of Moses, peace be upon them after they left Egypt as stated in the Holy Quran Since ancient times, fava beans have been used as a dietary alternative to meat, in addition to chickpeas, because they have a sufficient amount of protein that is essential to humans. It is also rich in dietary fiber and important minerals such as iron, zinc, magnesium, Potassium, copper, and also contains some acids that help to raise immunity within the body also helps to reduce cholesterol in the blood and fight cancer

## LENTILS

It is now known that 300 grams of lentils are equivalent to about 500 grams of red meat, and this is why the lentils were used as a food for the ancient Egyptians. It is famous in popular neighborhoods as the flesh of the poor

Lentils also contribute to lowering cholesterol, heart disease, and high pressure, as well as it contains a high proportion of folic acid, which reduces the risk of fetal deformity of the fetus

## CARROTS

Carrots were carved on the walls of the Pharaonic temples, where the ancient Egyptian used them in stomach and chest treatments. It was also said that women used it as one of the essential cosmetics for the safety and health of the skin. Recently research has discovered that the islands are rich in vitamin A, which is essential for the safety of the skin, Iron, magnesium, phosphorus, sodium, potassium. It is rich in carotene, which activates, stimulates the process of regeneration of tissues and cells. It is a useful process for removing wrinkles from the face, forehead and strengthening hair and nails.

Carrots contain dietary fibers that help prevent gastrointestinal disorder, constipation, improve vision, treat eye strain, reduce blood pressure, improve liver tissue, increase blood flow, prevent tooth decay

## OLIVE OIL

Ancient Egyptians attributed the credit of human learning to the cultivation of olives and the wisdom of the goddess Isis. The containers containing olive oil were found among the Egyptian tombs during the recent process of uncovering the statues.

Olive oil is resistant to strokes, heart attacks, excess cholesterol in the blood, reduces hunger, antioxidants, helps lower blood pressure, contains monounsaturated fats, many vitamins (A / K / D / E) In the elimination of constipation, increases the speed of digestion, eliminate ulcers and gastritis, get rid of gas and bloating, works to reduce the proportion of diabetes and prevention of gallstones disease and gallstones

## GARLIC AND ONIONS

The onion appeared in the Spring Festival food in the sixth family and was associated with the appearance of one of the legends of ancient Memphis, which tells that one of the kings of the ancient Egyptians had a single child and the little prince suffered a mysterious illness and the inability of doctors

Then one of the priests put the fruit of the onions under the head of the prince after reading some magical talismans and then breaking it at sunrise in the dawn and put it on the nose of the little prince to bite the juice and the healing of the Prince and the ancient Egyptians believed in the ability of the onion fruit to heal and became eating onions at sunrise omen The pharaohs believed that onions will remove the evil used to fill onions in cans and hang them in the entrances of houses or in places that can be seen from home. This is the tradition still practiced today by some Egyptians in the present era. A large area in the kitchen of ancient Egypt, was considered an activist must be taken care of in a sustainable manner and was an immature distribution to the workers every day to prevent them from diseases and workers were beating the work in the absence of garlic for them in the daily meal and the rate of eating garlic up to 10 beads a day with the rest of the components of the meal and indicate inscriptions on the walls of the temples Pharaonic that "garlic" a great place in the ancient Egyptians increased resistance to human diseases The immune system strengthens the longevity, and they call it the "antidote of the poor". Our ancestors used to make children's necklaces to protect against contagious diseases. It was eaten with radish to give the workers strength and activity. Scientific experiments have shown that they have anti-cancer medical properties. Garlic contains lysine, anti-bacterial, fungi, viruses, and oxidation. The antibiotic works well. The garlic can be taken to those who do not like it in the form of tablets or powder. Onion contains volatile oils, Fibers, organic acids (folic acid and pantothenic acid), metals such as sodium, potassium, calcium, magnesium, phosphorus, and also fights cancer, especially stomach cancer

## Lettuce

Pharaoh's doctors mentioned lettuce in medical papyrus, which was included in many treatments and appeared through engraving on the walls of temples that linked the god responsible for fertilization, reproduction, and lettuce by placing piles of lettuce under his feet.

The male stood in front of him to receive his help and advice in return for large quantities of lettuce, which means that lettuce treats the problem of ED in men also knows that it helps in digestion, strengthens the eyesight, and relieves the pain of menstruation, giving psychological comfort, it is known that the nutritional value of lettuce plant enriched with vitamin E is an enriched vitamin, the balance of sex hormones and increases its secretion. This supports the old medicine's usefulness in enhancing the sexual power and treatment of ancient Egyptians with infertility

# Chapter 5. Fruits

## Dates

Dates palm trees are one of the oldest trees known to ancient Egyptians and were interested in planting them. Palm is one of the oldest cultivated plants in Egypt, dates are a good food for the general public, and found quantities of dates, in the graves of many ancient Egyptians. The ancient Egyptians were eating new or dry dates in times of crisis. Disasters, used in filling some types of cakes. Dates are rich in iron, calcium, potassium, sodium, phosphorus, zinc, copper, sulfur, all of which are essential for the formation of blood cells and the activation of nerves and brain and heart functions. It also contains vitamin B complex, which calms the nerves, especially after stress. The vitality of the body and its immunity against diseases, vitamin A, which helps to see at night, strengthens the immune system and increases the prevention of the body from diseases, where it is characterized that many of its nutrients do not need to digest the sugars in it provide the body with strength, immunity, thermal energy in time Short compared to "meat" for example You need more time to supply the body energy and dates are characterized by a high proportion of amino acids needed to build cells of the body, Repair of antimicrobial and antimicrobial agents

Dates are mentioned in the medical papyrus of Hearst within the therapeutic prescriptions of bladder diseases, dysplasia, stomach, bowel, and constipation. In papyrus, dates and other parts of the palm have been mentioned in several recipes to treat certain diseases, such as pain prevention and vomiting prevention. To prevent vomiting, a mixture of dates, wheat grains, a cup of milk, sugar

## POMEGRANATE

The pomegranate tree in ancient Egyptians was considered a symbol of well-being and hope. The bark of the tree was used to treat tapeworms in the stomach, according to one of the oldest medical papyrus, called Ebers. Pomegranate husk was used in dyeing leather in yellow and pomegranate boiled in water for skin diseases., treatment of burns and tumors Inscriptions were found on the walls of the tomb of El Amarna hills in Upper Egypt, dating back to the days of Amenhotep IV, one of the kings of the 18th Dynasty, emphasizing the importance of pomegranate fruits and trees in those ancient eras

The historical papyrus indicates that the ancient Egyptians knew it as Armani, "Raman", and the best pomegranate is red pomegranate of dark color.

## FIGS

Used by the Pharaohs in the treatment of many diseases, including diseases of the digestive system and the richness of figs with magnesium helps to reduce stress and strengthen the heart and blood circulation Experts advise more orange juice with purified fig also helps drink to get rid of stress, and for diabetics who feel the desire to eat The dessert and doctor's instructions prevent them. Figs are the best solution for them and also helps in constipation as experts advise

Sprinkle five pieces of dried figs in a quarter liter of lukewarm water and leave at night and then drink the water the next day with a mixture of figs. The fig ingredients help to treat fatigue and loss of concentration which affects some especially early in the spring and the rich zinc fig makes them perfect in improving mood It is the food of philosophers, geniuses, thinkers, innovators, wrestlers, athletes and warriors because it is a food that gives energy and vitality to the body.

## WATERMELON

It was mentioned in the papyrus of "Ebers" and it was said that the word Buduka is the origin of the word watermelon and was said to have moved from Egypt to the Mediterranean

Watermelon contains antioxidants, especially lycopene, ascorbic acid, citrulline, also contains a large amount of potassium, manganese are two elements that help to reduce high blood, prevent atherosclerosis and also works to reduce the proportion of urea in the blood and thus helps to cleanse the kidneys, protect it from inflammation as it is diuretic, helps to get rid of toxic ammonia, help the body get rid of excess fluid

# CHAPTER 6. HERBS

## CUMMINS

Cumin is known in ancient Egypt, which was cultivated on many banks of the Nile and was presented as gifts to temples. Cumin in ancient papyrus came in more than 60 prescription Calcium is an important source of iron and magnesium and its benefits. Its oil is very important to massage the body. Helps eliminate abdominal gases. Cumin is used in the treatment of colic and gastrointestinal disorders. It is used in cooking with a distinctive flavor Antioxidant because the substances present in them are considered the strongest among all powerful anti-cancer antioxidants Protects against memory loss and protects the body from colds especially when you drink it with lemon and is useful in treating respiratory diseases such as asthma and bronchitis.

Very useful for diabetics helps to produce insulin and thus balances blood sugar Anemia is treated with iron The use of cumin water in the face wash three times a day preserves the freshness of the skin and its cleanliness

Accelerates the healing of wounds, sores and boils Iron found in latency helps maintain metabolism activity properly

Cumin works to increase the burning rate of your body especially if eaten every morning with ginger

Cumin fills the appetite and resists the desire to eat because it stimulates signs of satiety that reach the brain enough to eat a cup of honey in the morning Strengthens immunity

Cumin is healthy for women of all ages and is known for its effective effect on the menstrual cycle and also compensates for blood loss So you can take one cup of cumin mixed with lemon juice and honey to avoid any future problems

Useful for kidney health Cumin warm drink treats pharyngitis and throat

You can prepare the face mask by gently mixing turmeric and cumin 3: 1 to prepare the face peeling mask. Honey can be used instead of water to mix all ingredients. Use it on your face to dry completely.

The benefits of cumin for hair Use equal amounts of cumin oil and olive oil after bathing, and use it on your hair Or on the bald part of the head. This promotes hair growth as well as hair loss

## ANISE

The original place of anise Egypt, where scientists found the Plantae of aniseed in the graves of the eastern desert of the city of Taiba as mentioned Anise in the papyrus Pharaonic, such as Ebers papyrus, among several therapeutic recipes, the most important use of anise seeds with boiled water as a drink to treat stomach disorders, Urinary incontinence, gum pain, toothache, mouth lotion

## HIBISCUS

Ancient Egyptians cared about the cultivation of hibiscus and used its flowers in some treatment recipes such as the use of painkillers in the head, worms are expelled from the intestines, lowering blood pressure, stimulating the brain, nervous system, accelerating digestion, killing microbes and useful for those who want to lose weight, and relieve menstrual pain.

## LIQUORICE

In 1923, the roots of liquorice were found in the tomb of King Tutankhamun. This plant has a very important therapeutic value in ancient Egyptians. It was treated many diseases of the digestive system, liver, intestines, it is very effective in the treatment of stomach ulcers and this is what has been proven by recent research that liquorice contains the substance of glycerin, which helps to heal the ulcer stomach and intestines

## SEEDS OF FLAX

The pharaohs used flaxseed to treat hemorrhoids, according to papyrus Herst, while another medical papyrus reported that flaxseed was used to treat wounds, sores, eczema, baldness, infections and the benefits of these seeds. Prevention of cancer because it contains high levels of omega-3 fatty acids that inhibit the growth of cancer tumors have been shown to have a clear role in the prevention of breast cancer, it is better to use mature flaxseed seeds without mature seeds without excessive consumption

# CHAPTER 7. HONEY

Egypt was known in the Torah as the land of milk, honey and fertile soil with millions of beekeepers in its territory. Excavations in the tombs of the pharaohs revealed the containers of honey covered and retained aromatic smell,

The ancient Egyptian beekeepers were also known for their tours along the banks of the Nile during the four seasons to take flowers throughout the year. In ancient Pharaonic paintings, Pharaohs' love of the bees was seen as a symbol of the king who used the ancient Egyptians as honey in the food and gifts of the gods and also a material of important material in embalming

The most important evidence of this is the George Ebers Papyrus, where he gave a full description of the therapeutic properties of honey and the most important that "honey helps in the healing of wounds and in the treatment of gastrointestinal diseases and kidneys

Honey is a rich source of energy, which contains glucose and fructose, which promotes blood in the arteries quickly and is a great way to start the exercise and contains antioxidants that feed brain cells and promote memory, helps to reduce a cough during the winter months

Two tablespoons of honey are as effective as a sedative cough. Instead of resorting to hypnotics to treat insomnia, honey can be used. The sweetness of honey causes high levels of insulin in the blood, which in turn releases serotonin and then converts serotonin into melatonin, it is a chemical that helps to sleep.

Aphrodisiac honey and regular consumption of this spoon a day can promote sexual desire

# CHAPTER 8. IMPORTANT PRESCRIPTIONS IN ANCIENT EGYPTIANS

Medicine was one of the branches of knowledge that excelled in ancient Egypt and was followed by the development of ancient Pharaonic history, ranging from diagnosis of diseases and even the use of medicines in the treatment of ancient Egyptian has benefited from all available materials of plant or organic elements in the formation of various treatments for many diseases, Science took a lot of time, effort, observation and experience to the extent that it treated many diseases Many of the medicines used by ancient Egyptians relied heavily on plant elements. It was used to treat the pain of the head, where the ancient Egyptians extracted many medicines such as mint, coriander, wormwood, Saffron, celery, radish, flaxseed, pumpkin, pine, dates, cumin, dill, pomegranate, and other plants. Honey, cow's milk, goats, fish oil, bull liver, the oldest and most important documents recorded on diseases and symptoms and how to treat them, especially the use of plant medicines.

## DISINFECTANT RECIPES FOR INTESTINES

1 Soaked barley with the addition of barley grain, chickpea, and fresh sycamore and eat it.

2 Milk, Sycamore fruit, honey where the mixture is boiled, dried and eaten for four days.

## RECIPES TO GET RID OF ABDOMINAL PAIN

1 Desalination of wheat grain boiled honey to get rid of the pain.

2 A mixture of dates, honey and mulch and eaten

## RECIPE FOR IMPROVING APPETITE

1 Mix bread with honey and water and take to improve appetite.

## PRESCRIPTION AGAINST THE SCALY

1 Use the fermented, wet bread to put on the head to get rid of the crust.

## RECIPES FOR THE TREATMENT OF A COUGH

1 consists of milk cow fat and honey and feed the patient for four days.

2 dipped melon where it soaked in water and drank for four days as well as boiled watermelon with a barley drink and also drank for four days.

## RECIPE FOR TREATMENT OF INCONTINENCE

1 Boil a mixture of pine, groundnut, barley and filtered and taken on four days

## PRESCRIPTION FOR THE TREATMENT OF ED

1 Honey Bee 300 grams

2 Beef 2 grams

3 The grain of the pond 6 grams

4 Celery 4 grams.

5 Seeds of fennel 3 grams.

6 Seeds of dill 3 grams.

7 Clove 2 grams.

Mix all ingredients and take a tablespoon before each meal for at least 20 days

## RECIPE FOR HAIR BEAUTY

1 Oil of Perafin 60 ml.

2 Watercress seed oil 30 ml.

3 Castor oil 30 ml.

4 Olive oil 30 ml.

5 Almond oil 20 ml.

6 Coconut oil 20 ml.

7 Pomegranate oil 20 ml.

Mix all oils and put mix on hair once a day

## RECIPE FOR TREATING RESPIRATORY DISEASES

1 Thyme 40 g.

2 Coriander 40 g.

3 fenugreek 40 g.

4 Pomegranate 40 g.

5 Dill 30 g.

6 Cinnamon 30 g.

7 Carnation 20 g.

Mix the amount on each other and take a teaspoon on a glass of boiled water, honey and drink after eating 3 times a day for a month

# CHAPTER 9. AROMATHERAPY

Aromatherapy is an ancient means of healing, relaxation, and revitalization through the use of plants where the ancient Egyptians extracted herbs and aromatic oils substitute for medicines

## PEPPERMINT OIL

The Pharaohs used 3 or 4 drops of peppermint oil over a cup of boiling water to treat bronchitis, Elimination of bad breath, dental treatment, cold where inhaled through the nose as was used in mouthwash.

## CAMPHOR OIL

Use camphor extracts to treat asthma, cough, and allergies by massaging the chest area with five drops of oil before going to bed, as well as massage the front with 3 drops of oil for 3 minutes to treat nervous system disorders, migraines, open and clean the pores of the skin.

## SANDALWOOD

Ancient Egyptians used sandalwood mixed with parts of the eucalyptus tree to eliminate arthritis, muscle and sciatica by massage the area to be treated for 15 minutes three times a week, as well as to treat skin wrinkles by massage the body with honey and sandal milk for 20 minutes.

## LAVENDER FLOWER

The ancient Egyptians considered that massage the back part of the neck with 3 drops of lavender oil for 6 minutes helps relieve insomnia, snoring, and vertigo, as well as removing the flying insects from the body. It also helps to relax and sleep when you massage the body with 15 drops of lavender oil by spray

## ORANGE FLOWER

The orange blossom was used by ancient Egyptians to combat stress and a sense of optimism as well as bathing for further recovery and foot massage

## BERGAMOT OIL

Ancient Egyptians treated skin diseases such as psoriasis, eczema, acne, burns, black spots, rheumatism, rashes with bergamot oil once every night.

## AMBERGRIS

Pharaohs found that the use of amber fights depression, and provides better focus after adding two drops of oil in the hand and spread together and then inhale deeply

## FRANKINCENSE

The ancient Egyptians used frankincense to slow the rapid pulse of the heart, to meditate and to help the mind to pray. It is also one of the most important aromatic incense because it has profound benefits for increasing concentration, gaining calm, stopping chatter, raising morale,

## MYRRH

Myrrh was one of the most widely used oils in ancient Egypt because it has a permanent scent. It is used to raise awareness and give a strong boost to the feelings of indifference and weakness in addition to its ability to cool hot feelings and bear difficult conditions

## ALOE VERA

Ancient Egyptian efforts have concluded that cactus treats sunburn, skin pimples, insect bites, treatment of athlete's foot inflammation and dry skin allergies

## Clove Oil

To treat tooth pain, stop vomiting and reduce the desire to drink alcohol Pharaohs used water mixed with 3 drops of clove oil to relieve pain

## Black Seeds Oil

The efforts of the pharaohs did not stop at the outer body, but their discoveries in the medical sciences developed into oils to contain the internal organs. They used black seeds oil to reduce cholesterol, treat parasitic infections, treat gastrointestinal infections of diarrhea, colic, stomach pain, treat indigestion and strengthen the immune system. A Daily dose of 4 drops on any drink

## Watercress Oil

The ancient Egyptians found that the watercress oil contributes to the fight against diabetes with the increase of sexual activity in men when placing five drops on any drink once a day as treated by hair loss and strengthen the follicles to prevent early baldness by massage the scalp with some droplets and then wash the hair after 15 minutes

## Sesame oil

Sesame oil comes for weight gain, supplemental feeding and eliminating menstrual pain. It is also considered a mild laxative and protects the arteries from stiffness

## Onion oil

Onion oil is a natural tonic and antibiotic that reduces the level of sugar in the blood and prevents liver disorder if you put a small spoon of oil on a hot drink as a daily dose, as well as it is used to prevent cracks of the breast, killing germs and remove pimples with a small spoon of oil on warm water to massage the affected area

# Chapter 10. Face And Skin Care

In Ancient Egypt, the pharaohs invented natural ways to care for the skin, using Aloe Vera gel and dry sand to open the pores of the skin and remove impurities cactus plant is one of the most important elements that the queen used to soften the skin, heal wounds, and treat minor burns.

The next time you decide to spend a day on the beach, you can take advantage of the ancient Egyptian way of foot treatment so that you can mix dry sand with cactus gel and rub your feet and focus particularly on areas experiencing drought problems

## RECIPE FOR THE TREATMENT OF DRY SKIN PROBLEMS

1 Two tablespoons of canola oil

2 Three tablespoons of dry beach sands

3 3 to 5 points of rosemary oil

Mix all ingredients in an empty container and rub the areas with problems and wash them

## ALMOND OIL

The ancient Egyptians used almond oil and added it to cosmetics and perfumes. It later became clear that the oil is beneficial for the skin. It moisturizes the dry skin, treats the wrinkles of the skin and of course it is also one of the secrets behind the beauty of Queen Cleopatra's flawless skin The benefits of many almond oil can be easily found in the markets and it is rich in vitamins and minerals

## RECIPE BY ALMOND OIL FOR NATURAL SKIN

1 A glass of almond oil

2 8 points of concentrated rose oil

3 Half a cup of rose water

4 Half a cup of distilled water

5 4 tablespoons of beeswax

Mix the water with the honey and let them homogenize in the mixer at low speed and gradually add almond oil, rose water and the rest of the mixture will be a rigid and dense mixture, then put it in a jar and use it when needed

## HONEY AND MILK

Queen like Cleopatra bathed in milk because it is rich in lactic acid, which Peeling the skin and renews its youth

Queen Cleopatra is famous for her beautiful skin and one of the secrets of her cosmetic treatments is the milk and honey bath that is still used to help clean the deep layers of the skin.

## HONEY AND MILK BATH FOR QUEEN CLEOPATRA

1 Half a cup of fresh milk

2 Half a cup of honey

3 Two tablespoons of Jojoba oil tea

Mix the ingredients in a large bowl and place in a warm bath and leave on your skin for up to 20 minutes

In order to benefit the skin of its useful components, this recipe is enough for one bath

## ALOE VERA TO CLEAN THE SKIN

Cleopatra was not only the most intelligent and powerful Egyptian woman, but she was also the most attractive. One of the ingredients that accompanied her in her daily routine was aloe vera that used to unify the skin and remove the accumulated dirt on the surface of the skin. Now used in the production of cosmetics for skin care because of its importance in moisturizing and purifying the skin It is best to use it before sleeping to sleep by placing an aloe leaf on a piece of cotton and wipe your face completely.

## SEA SALT FOR SKIN PEELING

Sea salt is known for its great benefits to the body because it contains a mineral extract capable of restoring youth to the skin and fighting many skin problems. The queen used raw sea salt to give her a soft, clean skin

For the use of sea salt in skin peeling

Mix cup olive oil, cup sweet almond oil and a few points of any essential oil and rub the skin and body to remove dead cells and leave the skin more freshness

## AVOCADO TO GET RID OF PUFFY EYES

Rich in fatty acids and vitamins have long been using masks made of avocados to nourish skin and hair and are eaten this fruit is useful for the body at home and abroad. If you want to follow the method of Egyptology in ancient Egypt to get rid of swelling under the eyes can be placed mashed avocados every day before sleep until healing

## APPLE CIDER VINEGAR

One of the most common skin care methods in ancient Egyptian civilization is vinegar, which was used to wash the skin because it stimulates blood circulation and regulates the acidity of the skin. To make a vinegar solution you need a plate of warm water to add a quarter cup of apple cider vinegar then wash your skin first, then wash your face with a mixture of apple cider vinegar and let your skin dry off on its own

# CHAPTER 11. MEDICAL PAPYRUS DISCOVERED

## EDWIN SMITH PAPYRUS

Edwin Smith, an American researcher who visited the Egyptian city of Luxor and lived there for a long time. In 1862, an Egyptian merchant named Mustafa Agha appeared to sell the papyrus. It was purchased by Edwin Smith, who was the first to reveal her medical condition and remained in possession until his death. In 1930, Dr. James Henry translated papyrus and printed the first translated version of English. In 1938, the papyrus was moved to the Brooklyn Museum. In 1948, the papyrus was transferred to the New York Academy of Medicine, papyrus is written in hieroglyphics and is considered by the researchers and specialists as the oldest and first medical document in the history of mankind. Some Egyptian archaeologists expect the author to be Egyptian doctor Amenhotep. Papyrus paper describes anatomical observations, applied surgery, examination, diagnosis and treatment for more than 48 types of diseases in detail

Among the treatments described are a closure of wounds, treatment of paralysis, spinal cord injuries, prevention of infection, treatment using honey, rotten bread, and talk of stopping bleeding using raw meat

## EBERS PAPYRUS

The name of the papyrus belongs to Mr. George Ebers, who purchased it from Luxor city and translated it in 1875, length of 20 meters and a width of 30 centimeters it contains has many medical methods for the treatment of eye diseases, surgery, anatomy, internal medicine, and skin. The papyrus also provides a recipe for helping to grow hair in the bald head using the Scales of some reptiles like crocodiles, Among the diseases recorded by the papyrus is rash and provided several recipes for the manufacture of ointments.

## HEARST PAPYRUS

The Hearst Papyrus is a medical kingdom consisting of 18 pages containing approximately 260 paragraphs. It includes parts of the digestive system, urinary system, teeth, bones, and hair, as well as therapeutic recipes for some unspecified diseases.It also includes some Magic spells and the seeds of anise as a drink for the treatment of gastric ulcers and dyspnea.

## CHESTER BEATTY PAPYRUS

The papyrus is given by the businessman Sir Alfred Beattie to the British Museum after found during the excavations in the village of the workers of the cemeteries. This 19 papyrus were scattered in different places, including the Ashmolean Museum in Oxford, the

French Institute in Cairo and the Chester Museum Beate in Dublin While the third part of the Papyrus contains magical cures for the treatment of migraine headaches and the sixth part papyrus most of the paragraphs revolve around anal diseases, while her background carries little prescriptions with many magical spells for unknown diseases.

## BERLIN PAPYRUS

The papyrus was discovered in the Saqqara region and then sold to Friedrich Wilhelm king of Prussia in 1827 and deposited in the Berlin Museum. The method of writing refers to her belonging to the nineteenth family. The papyrus treats breast diseases and presents methods of contraception and testing to determine the sex of the fetus (male or female),  The Berlin Papyrus one of the few medical papyri that has treated any of one of the disorders of the nervous system describes the papyrus case of paralysis of the facial nerve, which usually affects one side of the face and provides for evaporation of the patient says evaporation to rid him of paralysis of one side of his face as well as the side of his mouth.

## RAMESSEUM PAPYRUS

Ramesseum papyrus was discovered in 1896, where 17 the papyrus was found inside a wooden box at the bottom of a tomb behind the Great Ramesseum Temple in the city of Thebes. One of them referred to Pharaoh Amenemhat III of the 12th Dynasty. The medical part of the Ramesseum papyrus is located in the third, fourth and fifth papyrus, fourth part also contains prescriptions for gynecology and children, while the fifth papyrus includes medical concepts, treatments for muscle and tendon injuries, as well as magic spells.

## BROOKLYN PAPYRUS

The papyrus treats snake bites only and is kept in the Brooklyn Museum and dates back to the 1930s or perhaps the beginning of the Ptolemaic era. The upper part of the papyrus contains the classification of different types of snakes, their bites up to 38. The following section includes an overview of the drugs used to get rid of snake venom and how to expel them, close their mouths and some magic spells that are used to cure snake bites The onion has a special place in this papyrus in the cases of snake bites. It is well mixed in a barley drink to cause vomiting. In another section, the onion should be in the hands of a priest wherever he goes because it eliminates the venom of any male or female snake. If the onion is mixed with barley juice and poured throughout the house on New Year's Day, no snake can enter the house.

# About the Author

**Mohamed Malah** was born in a small town called el kanater, Egypt, Graduated from the Faculty of Law, Cairo University 2007, He is reading in various fields especially literature, history, He loves moving between cities and getting to know the secrets of ancient Egyptian civilization inside Egypt, passionate about the mysteries of history and ancient civilizations.

www.ingramcontent.com/pod-product-compliance
Lightning Source LLC
Chambersburg PA
CBHW061541250726

48657CB00006B/2275